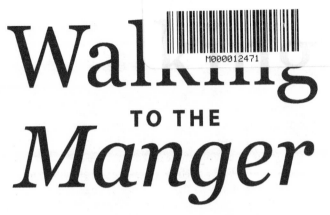

Walking

TO THE

Manger

Four Weeks of Daily
Devotions for Advent

Butch Odom

Healthy Living
for Church and Home
✦RESOURCES FROM CHURCH HEALTH

Founded in 1987, Church Health is a charitably funded, faith-based not-for-profit organization that provides comprehensive, high-quality, affordable health care to working underserved people and their families and gives people tools to live healthier lives. With the generous support of volunteer providers, the faith community, donors and community partners, we work tirelessly to improve health and well-being so that people can experience the full richness of life. For more information visit www.ChurchHealth.org.

The mission of Church Health is to reclaim the church's biblical commitment to care for our bodies and spirits.

Walking to the Manger: Four Weeks of Daily Devotions for Advent
© 2013, 2019 Church Health Center, Inc. Memphis, TN

ISBN: 978-1-62144-064-2

Healthy Living for Church and Home brings you practical tools and insights to help you faithfully create habits to honor God and know fullness of life.

Cover and interior design: Lizy Heard
Image: © pingebat / Adobe Stock

To my favorite author, illustrator, drummer and lawyer, my sister Linda Odom, and her loving family, husband John and children Lillian and Eric.

Our Mission

Church Health is a faith-based organization. The mission of Church Health is to reclaim the church's biblical commitment to care for our bodies and spirits. Each day, we stand ready to care for people who are hurting but live within a health care system that has left them behind.

We know from history that Christians have always cared for the underserved, both in body and spirit. Jesus asks us to care about what he cares about—wellness and wholeness of all people.

In Memphis, Tennessee, Church Health provides clinical services to working underserved individuals in the areas of medical, dental, optometry, physical rehabilitation, and behavioral health, along with wellness services in nutrition, life health coaching, child well-being, and disease prevention. Our funding comes from charitable sources, and hundreds of volunteers augment our staff to care for thousands of patients. Beyond Memphis, we reach across the country and around the globe with a ministry of faith community nurses and publications for healthy living.

Your purchase and use of this publication shares in our mission to care for bodies and spirits in a way that shows the love and hope of Jesus on the road to living in healthier ways that honor God's love for us.

For more information visit www.ChurchHealth.org.

Introduction

Advent is the start, the arrival, the dawn of a journey that leads us not only to the manger where we find the Christ-child, but to a new understanding of our relationship to the world and to one another as people of faith. Advent is a journey in which the traveling is as full of lessons as the destination. As such, the season is a journey of faith.

An enduring traditional image of the Christmas story for me is Mary sitting on her donkey being led by Joseph, who is walking. Walking was as integral to the lives of Mary, Joseph and later Jesus as cars are to us. I am drawn to the discipline of walking as a way to connect Scripture to our lives in a tangible way.

The following collection of devotionals is designed to help you focus your thoughts for a few minutes each day during Advent. Advent Scriptures offered for daily reflection often give us a lens of physical or metaphorical movement toward each other and toward God. As this is a journey, I hope you will consider walking daily as a symbolic discipline of your Advent journey.

How to Use

E very week of reflections begins with a psalm and the opportunity to set a "movement goal," or a reasonable physical challenge for yourself. Your movement goal may be taking more steps each day, going for a daily walk, wearing a pedometer to count the distance you walk each day, or any other challenge you wish to set for yourself.

Each day offers a passage of Scripture along with a thought and a prayer. You may read any time during the day, or you may reflect on them while engaged in your chosen physical activity. Each page includes journal space for you to track the progress toward your goals and note any personal challenges or successes.

As you walk toward the Christ-child through the words of the prophets and the apostles, we pray that you may become healthier in body and spirit. May you be blessed while walking to the manger.

Visions of Advent

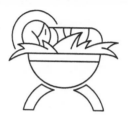

Restore us, O LORD God of hosts;
let your face shine, that we may be saved.
—Psalm 80:19

Movement Goal

....

....

....

Sunday

For a child has been born for us, a son given to us;
authority rests upon his shoulders;
and he is named
Wonderful Counselor, Mighty God,
Everlasting Father, Prince of Peace.

—Isaiah 9:6

Wonderful counselors do more listening than talking. As you begin your Advent journey, whether walking or sitting quietly and meditating, talk to God openly and honestly.

Gracious God, hear my prayers for guidance
throughout my Advent journey with you.
Amen.

Personal Reflection

....

....

....

Monday

*O that you would tear open the heavens
and come down, so that the mountains
would quake at your presence.*

—Isaiah 64:1

Advent—a time when Christians anticipate God moving toward us to dwell among us through Jesus, a time when we move toward God with intentionality. It is a time of hope as well as preparation as we walk to the manger together.

*Creator God, while I await your return
I am doing my part to try to build
the world you want. Be with me in
this daily journey to follow your will.
Amen.*

Personal Reflection

Tuesday

Yet, O LORD, you are our Father;
we are the clay, and you are our potter;
we are all the work of your hand.
Do not be exceedingly angry, O LORD
and do not remember iniquity forever.
Now consider, we are all your people.

—Isaiah 64:8–9

I love the imagery of the potter and clay. There is both an intimacy and messiness between the potter and clay. Yet the intimacy can move through the messiness to bring us—and make us—something of immeasurable beauty.

Creator God, open my heart and mind to you
so that I can become the person into which
you would mold me.
Amen.

Personal Reflection

....

....

....

Wednesday

He shall judge between the nations,
and shall arbitrate for many peoples;
they shall beat their swords into plowshares,
and their spears into pruning hooks ...

—Isaiah 2:4

In Isaiah's vision, tools of war are turned into farm implements and tools of destruction are turned into tools of creation—tools used to create food, sustenance. What a picture of the transformative power of God.

Sustainer God, open my eyes
to the hunger in my neighbor's eyes,
and give me the strength and wisdom to help.
Amen.

Personal Reflection

....

....

....

Thursday

God is faithful; by him you were called into the
fellowship of his Son, Jesus Christ our Lord.

—1 Corinthians 1:9

"God is faithful" is short and simple, but isn't it powerful? Wherever we are on our journey, God is loyal, devoted and trustworthy. God is dependable and dedicated. God is true and authentic.

Steadfast God, I give you thanks
for the many blessings you have bestowed on me.
Continue to nudge me to be
the person you want me to be.
Amen.

Personal Reflection

....

....

....

Friday

*... nation shall not lift up sword against nation,
neither shall they learn war any more.*

—Isaiah 2:4

Isaiah shares a radical vision of peace in God's coming kingdom when nations no longer learn war. Advent is a time to dream big dreams and to envision that time when God's kingdom is a reality and we walk in God's peace.

*Loving God, as your hands and feet on the earth,
make me a better peacemaker.
Amen.*

Personal Reflection

....

....

....

Saturday

Make me to know your ways, O LORD;
teach me your paths.

—Psalm 25:4

You have started a journey this week. Whether your walk has been physical, metaphorical or a mixture of both, you have been engaged in a conversation with God to help draw you closer to God's plan for you. Rejoice today in your progress, even if it seems insignificant.

God of wonder, you can make the faith
of a mustard seed do amazing things.
Continue walking beside me
as I continue in my journey toward you.
Amen.

Personal Reflection

Preparing the Way

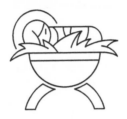

Righteousness will go before him, and will make a path for his steps.
—Psalm 85:13

Movement Goal

....

....

....

Sunday

Comfort, O comfort my people,
says your God ... A voice cries out:
"In the wilderness prepare the way of the LORD,
make straight in the desert a highway for our God."

—Isaiah 40:1, 3

We live in a violent world where people commit heinous acts toward one another. And yet, as God's hands and feet working and walking in the world, we are called to comfort one another, to embrace the vision of this passage and work at preparing the way of the Lord.

Loving God, help me be a better voice of your will,
of your message, of your peace.
Amen.

Personal Reflection

Monday

"Every valley shall be lifted up,
and every mountain and hill made low;
the uneven ground shall become level,
and the rough places a plain.
Then the glory of the Lord shall be revealed,
and all people shall see it together,
for the mouth of the Lord has spoken."

—Isaiah 40:4–5

Have you ever walked in mud, loose gravel or a dry, sandy beach and noticed how quickly you get tired? Are there people in your life whose faith is like walking on loose gravel? Pray for guidance so that you can help them find firmer footing.

Almighty God, be with me in my personal efforts to
make uneven ground level for others.
Amen.

Personal Reflection

....

....

....

Tuesday

Faithfulness will spring up from the ground,
and righteousness will look down from the sky.
The LORD will give what is good,
and our land will yield its increase.
Righteousness will go before him,
and will make a path for his steps.

—Psalm 85:11–13

The psalmist provides a beautiful image of God's coming peaceable kingdom. As you walk today, imagine what faithfulness would look like in your neighborhood if it were to spring up from the ground.

God of peace, speak to me
so I can be the peacemaker you want me to be.
Amen.

Personal Reflection

....

....

....

Wednesday

*"And you, child, will be called
the prophet of the Most High;
for you will go before the Lord to prepare his ways,
to give knowledge of salvation to his people
by the forgiveness of their sins."*

—Luke 1:76–77

These words came from Zechariah in dedicating his son, John the Baptist, to the Lord. As you walk through your day, consider how you prepare the way for the Lord by your words and actions.

*Understanding God, give me strength and wisdom
to be a better herald of your coming kingdom.
Amen.*

Personal Reflection

....

....

....

Thursday

*Now John wore clothing of camel's hair
with a leather belt around his waist,
and his food was locusts and wild honey.*

—Matthew 3:4

It is hard to imagine believing someone like John who is shouting, "Christ is coming!" As people of faith, we are challenged to remember that God can and often does use unlikely people to carry God's message forward. We have the opportunity to do the same with each step we take.

*Loving, understanding God, help me to see your
light in all the people who cross my path today.
Amen.*

Personal Reflection

....

....

....

Friday

[John the Baptist] went into all the regions around the Jordan, proclaiming a baptism of repentance for the forgiveness of sins, as it is written in the book of the words of the prophet Isaiah, "The voice of one crying out in the wilderness: 'Prepare the way of the Lord, make his paths straight.'"

—Luke 3:3–4

If time and weather permit, consider changing the location of your walk today. Walk a new path and imagine you are John the Baptist walking in the wilderness. How does your life proclaim, "Prepare the way of the Lord?"

Gracious God, thank you for giving strength to my voice so that I can better proclaim your truth.
Amen.

Personal Reflection

Saturday

I thank my God every time I remember you,
constantly praying with joy
in every one of my prayers for all of you,
because of your sharing in the gospel
from the first day until now.

—Philippians 1:3–5

In important part of Paul's prayer life was to offer prayers of thanksgiving for the work of other people of faith. Consider people of faith who help you move forward in your faith walk, and offer a prayer of thanks to God for them.

Loving God, for those people around me whose
lives shine as a beacon directing me to your truth,
I give you thanks.
Amen.

Personal Reflection

....

....

....

WEEK 3
Personal Preparation

Then our mouth was filled with laughter,
and our tongue with shouts of joy;
then it was said among the nations,
"The LORD has done great things for them."
—Psalm 126:2

Movement Goal

Sunday

*The spirit of the Lord G*OD *is upon me,*
*because the L*ORD *has anointed me;*
he has sent me to bring good news to the oppressed,
to bind up the brokenhearted,
to proclaim liberty to the captives,
and release to the prisoners;
*to proclaim the year of the L*ORD*'s favor,*
and the day of vengeance of our God;
to comfort all who mourn.

—Isaiah 61:1–2

This is a wonderful image of the movement of God in our world to reflect on as we begin our week. God: our healer, our liberator, and our comforter who turns sorrow to joy.

Gracious God, open my heart
so that you can work within me at all times.
Amen.

Personal Reflection

....

....

....

Monday

... to provide for those who mourn in Zion—
to give them a garland instead of ashes,
the oil of gladness instead of mourning,
the mantle of praise instead of a faint spirit.
They will be called oaks of righteousness,
the planting of the LORD, to display his glory.

—Isaiah 61:3

I grew up in a lakeside community known as Keuka Park, New York, home of Keuka College. The motto of Keuka was: "Mighty oaks from little acorns grow." It is so easy to feel insignificant in this world, but Isaiah reminds us of the transforming significance we have as a gift from God.

Loving God, help me to realize the potential
you see in me.
Amen.

Personal Reflection

Tuesday

May the God of peace himself sanctify you entirely; and may your spirit and soul and body be kept sound and blameless at the coming of our Lord Jesus Christ.

—1 Thessalonians 5:23

The connection between faith and health is mysterious. Yet, this verse reminds us that being holy requires attention to our bodies and our spirits. As you walk today, consider how the movement benefits your spirit as well as your body.

*God of peace, help make me
a sacred instrument of your will.
Amen.*

Personal Reflection

....

....

....

Wednesday

I will deal with all your oppressors at that time.
And I will save the lame and gather the outcast,
and I will change their shame into praise
and renown in all the earth.

—Zephaniah 3:19

Everyone comes in contact with outcasts, even if the outcast in your life is just the awkward and insecure person who makes people uncomfortable whenever he or she is around. Do you interact with such people in positive ways or do you help add to their feelings of separation?

Understanding God, help me see your imprint
on each person I see this day.
Amen.

Personal Reflection

....

....

....

Thursday

On that day it shall be said to Jerusalem:
Do not fear, O Zion;
do not let your hands grow weak.

—Zephaniah 3:16

Whether you are praying or helping a neighbor, your hands are an important element in your service to God and others. If you can do so without causing pain, make a fist as tight as you are able, then spread your fingers as wide as you can. Repeat this several times throughout the day as a reminder of serving God and others in ordinary ways.

Gracious God, I thank you today
for hands that can serve you in a variety of ways.
Amen.

Personal Reflection

....

....

....

Friday

Surely God is my salvation;
I will trust, and will not be afraid,
for the LORD GOD is my strength and my might;
he has become my salvation.
With joy you will draw water
from the wells of salvation.

—Isaiah 12:2–3

Imagine a time when you were very thirsty, maybe even dehydrated. As you begin to sip on water, you feel your body coming back into balance. When you drink water today, think of how this is a wonderful metaphor of our salvation.

Creator God, thank you for life-giving water
that quenches the thirst of my spirit.
Amen.

Personal Reflection

....

....

....

Saturday

*And the crowds asked [John the Baptist],
"What then should we do?" In reply he said to
them, "Whoever has two coats must share with
anyone who has none; and whoever has food must
do likewise."*

—Luke 3:10–11

You are approaching a season of gift giving. Consider taking this passage literally. Take a few moments to clean out your closet of gently used clothing or your pantry of food you won't use. If you do not know a family in need, share these items with a local church, clothes closet or food pantry.

*Merciful God, in this season of giving,
help me be mindful of the needs
of my brothers and sisters.
Amen.*

Personal Reflection

WEEK 4

Unlikely People, Extraordinary Choices

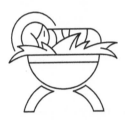

Light dawns for the righteous,
and joy for the upright in heart.
—Psalm 97:11

Movement Goal

....

....

....

Sunday

*Now, therefore thus you shall say to my servant
David: Thus says the LORD of hosts:
I took you from the pasture, from following the
sheep to be prince over my people Israel.*

—2 Samuel 7:8

Today we are reminded that David, the youngest son, the lowly shepherd, was chosen by God to be king of the people of Israel. Likewise, God can work through you, as unlikely as you think you might be.

*God of mystery, help me hear your will
so that I can be the person you know I can be.
Amen.*

Personal Reflection

....

....

....

Monday

In the sixth month the angel Gabriel was sent by God to a town in Galilee called Nazareth, to a virgin engaged to a man whose name was Joseph, of the house of David. The virgin's name was Mary. And he came to her and said, "Greetings, favored one! The Lord is with you."

—Luke 1:26–28

It is an incredible gift to have God communicate so clearly as in this passage. For most of our faith journeys, we get a sense, sometimes vague, of what we think is God's will, and we then live into that sense. These verses remind us that God is with us even in confusing times.

Merciful God, thank you for being with me this and every day. Continue to guide me as I seek to do your will.
Amen.

Personal Reflection

....

....

....

Tuesday

Now the birth of Jesus the Messiah took place this way. When his mother Mary had been engaged to Joseph, but before they lived together, she was found to be with child from the Holy Spirit. Her husband Joseph, being a righteous man and unwilling to expose her to public disgrace, planned to dismiss her quietly.

—Matthew 1:18–19

Joseph's choice is often downplayed while Mary's obedience takes center stage. Joseph was going to deal with Mary's pregnancy in a gentle way for his time. After hearing an angel and taking a leap of faith, in his own obedience Joseph chose to remain at Mary's side and embrace his role as father of Jesus.

Gracious God, give me ears to hear your voice so I can make decisions that are more informed by you. Amen.

Personal Reflection

....

....

....

Wednesday

But when the fullness of time had come,
God sent his Son, born of a woman, born under the
law, in order to redeem those who were under the
law, so that we might receive adoption as children.

—Galatians 4:4–5

We can imagine young Mary looking down from atop her donkey and saying, "Joseph! It's time." She then gave birth to a child of great promise in the most humble of places, a manger. Nothing is impossible with God.

God of promise, many children will be born today,
some in settings as humble as your Son's.
Be with all parents so they may see
the promise in their children that you see.
Amen.

Personal Reflection

....

....

....

Thursday

The light shines in the darkness,
and the darkness did not overcome it.

—John 1:5

This is the season when we celebrate that night a star guided the world to the light wrapped in swaddling clothes and lying in a humble manger—God among us as a baby.

Holy God, thank you for sending a light into this
world to pierce the darkest places.
Amen.

Personal Reflection

Friday

*When they had finished everything required by the
law of the Lord, they returned to Galilee, to their
own town of Nazareth. The child grew and became
strong, filled with wisdom, and the favor of God
was upon him.*

—Luke 2:39–40

I wish more was known about the childhood of
Jesus. What games did he like to play? Did he show
consideration to his friends at an early age? The growth
of Jesus through normal stages of life affirms that
we also learn and grow as we move through our life
seasons.

*God of wonder, I offer a special prayer today
for all children. Help me nurture the children in my
life as you want me to do.
Amen.*

Personal Reflection

....

....

....

Saturday

Now after they had left, an angel of the Lord appeared to Joseph in a dream and said, "Get up, take the child and his mother, and flee to Egypt, and remain there until I tell you; for Herod is about to search for the child, to destroy him."

—Matthew 2:13

In these early verses of Matthew 2, Joseph listens to and takes the advice of angels three times. As this journey through Advent comes to a close, remember the faith of Mary and Joseph, an unlikely couple called to an extraordinary task.

Understanding God,
give me the faith of Mary and Joseph
so that I can do extraordinary things for you.
Amen.

Personal Reflection

....

....

....

Notes

Notes

Journey toward a healthier Easter

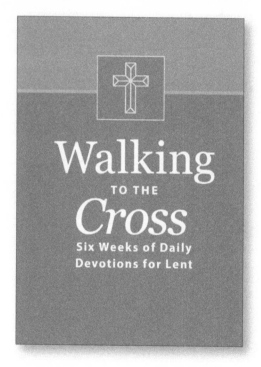

Daily reflections give us a lens for metaphorical movement toward God and healthier habits. In Walking to the Cross, *six weeks of devotions invite you to make reflecting, movement, and prayer a part of your daily Lenten practice.*

CPSIA information can be obtained
at www.ICGtesting.com
Printed in the USA
LVHW091040211119
638095LV00001B/130/P

9 781621 440642